Rico Eats a RAINBOW

DEDICATION

This book is dedicated to my nephew, Rico Jumper,
who has a beautiful appetite for learning new things.

and

In honor of my aunt, Bettye Lou Robinson.
I wish you could have read my book with your students.

Rico Eats a RAINBOW

Written By
Jessica M. Miller

Illustrated By
Sameer Kassar

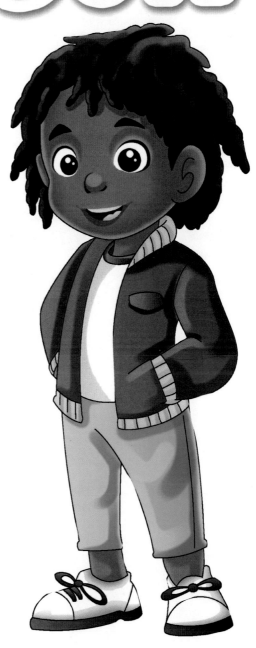

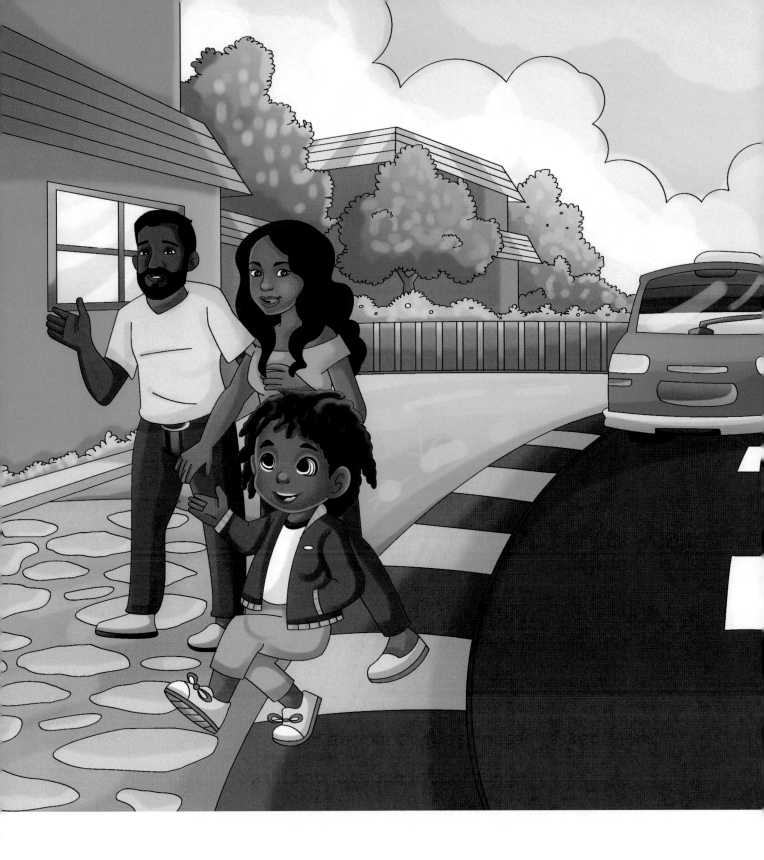

"Hi Rico. Did you have fun at your auntie's house?" asked Mom.

"Yes! I had lots and lots of fun!"

"What did you do at Auntie's house?" asked Dad.

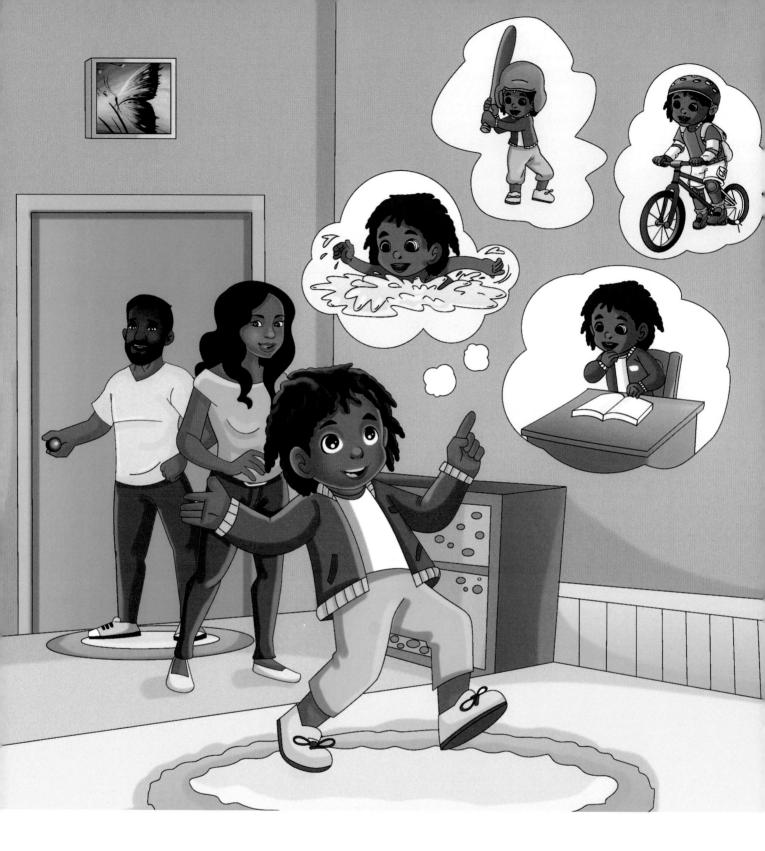

"We played outside and we went swimming," answered Rico.

"We rode our bicycles."

"We read books too."

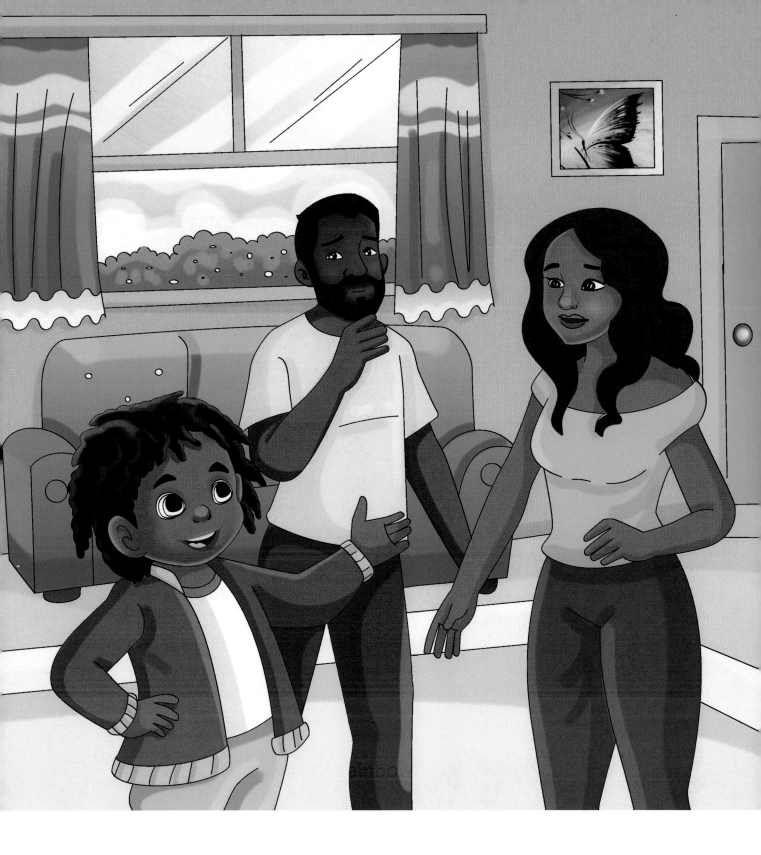

"And I ate a rainbow!" said Rico.

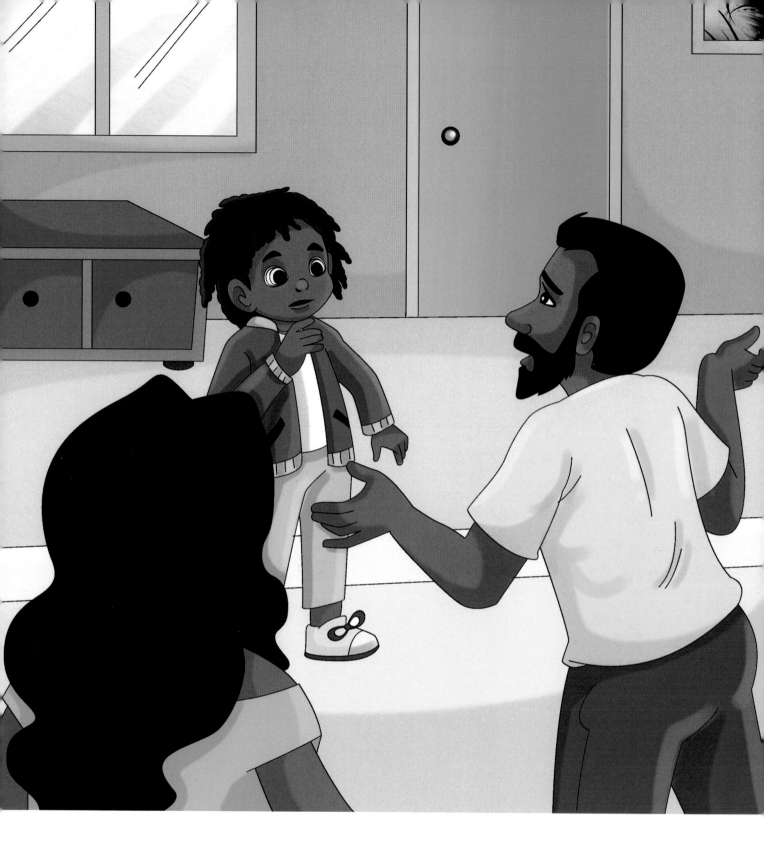

"You did WHAT?" asked Mom.

"Your auntie is always up to something," laughed Dad.

"Why did you eat a rainbow, son?"

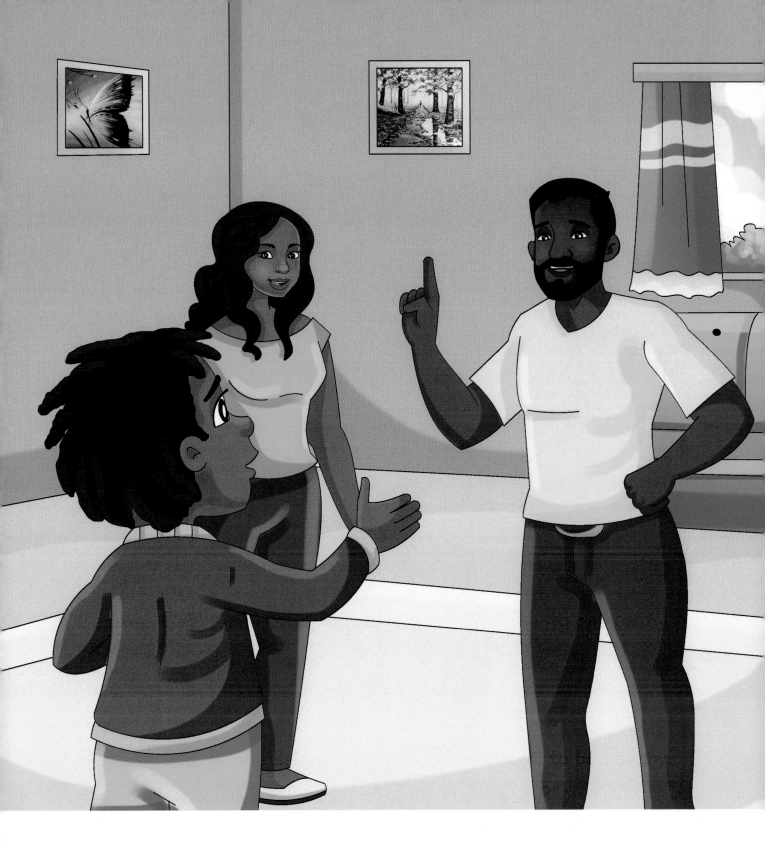

"Because Dad, Auntie said you have to eat a rainbow to be healthy."

"Really? How does a rainbow taste, son?"

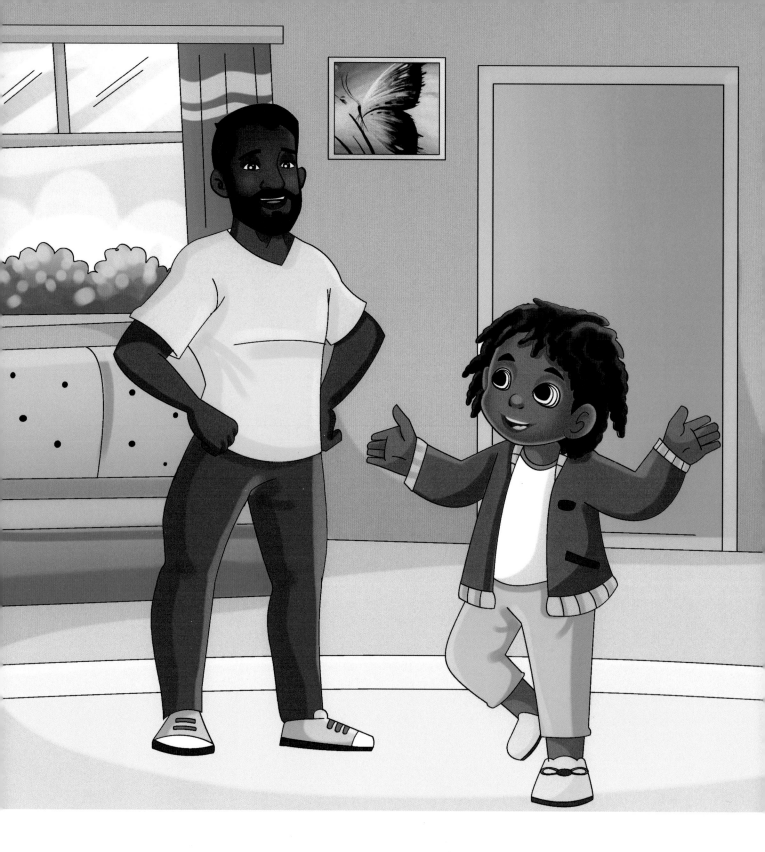

"Give me a break, Dad. I didn't eat a REAL rainbow!"

"To be healthy you have to eat all of the colors
of the rainbow," said Rico.

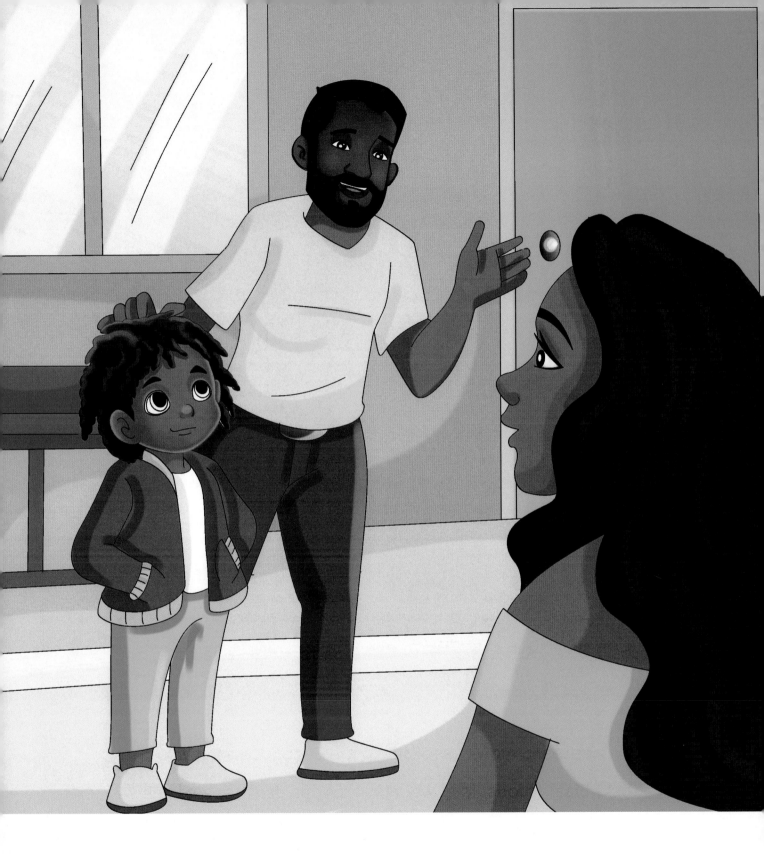

"Oh! That sounds like a great idea," Mom cheered.

"I want to see what eating a rainbow is all about," said Dad.

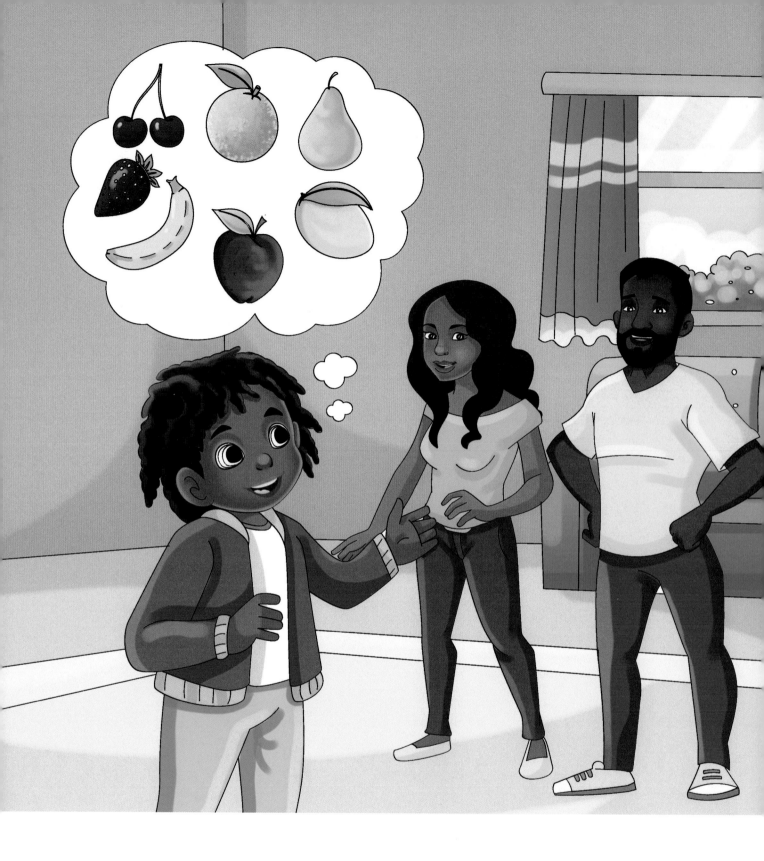

"We can find different foods in all of the colors
of the rainbow at the Farmers' Market,"
Rico told his parents.

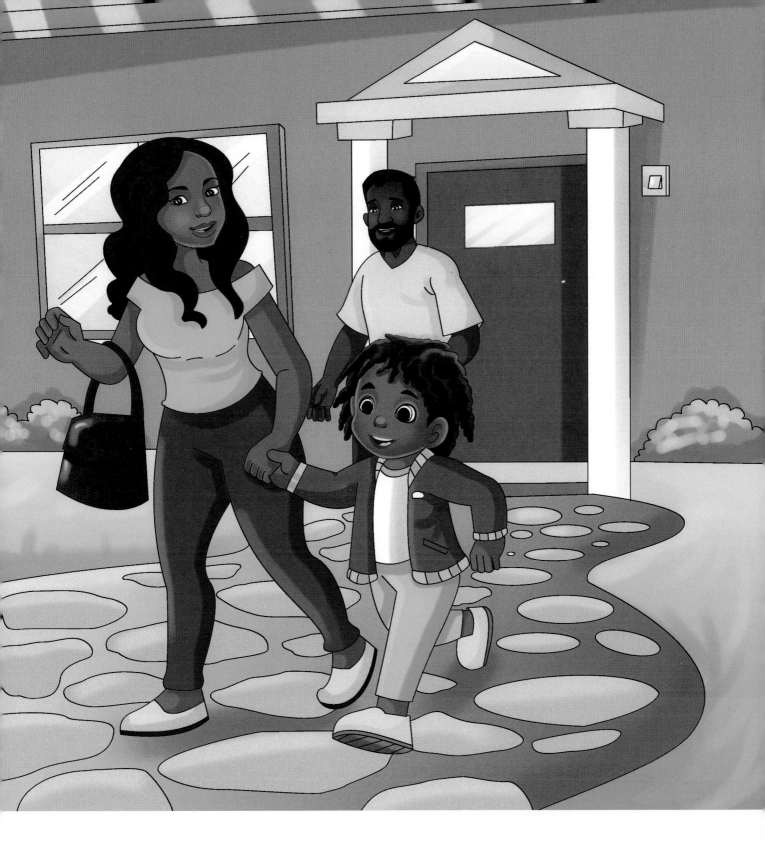

"Great! Let's take a walk to the Farmers' Market," said Mom.

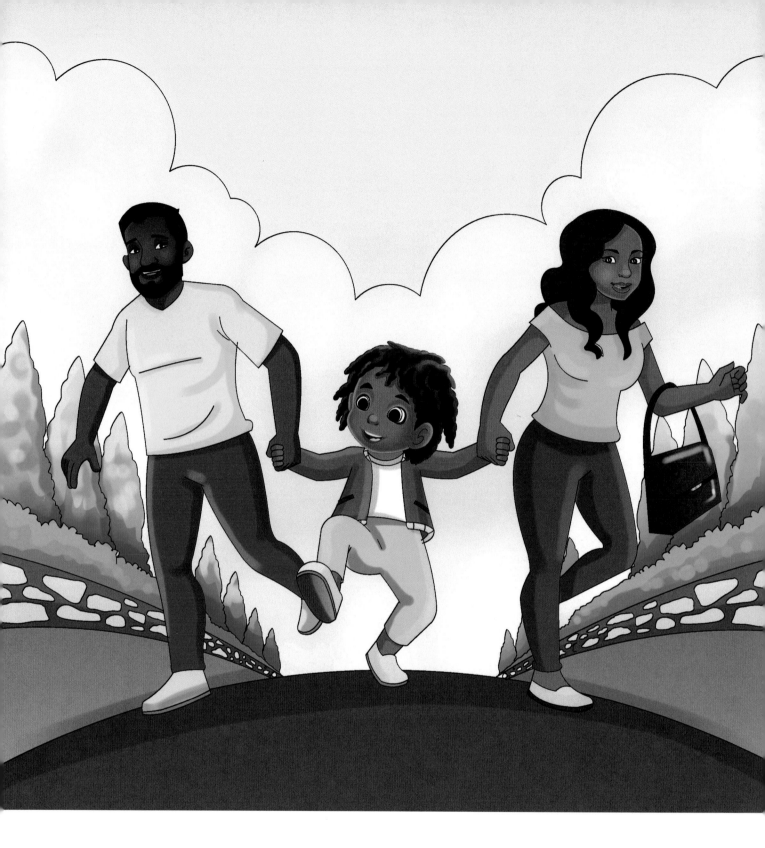

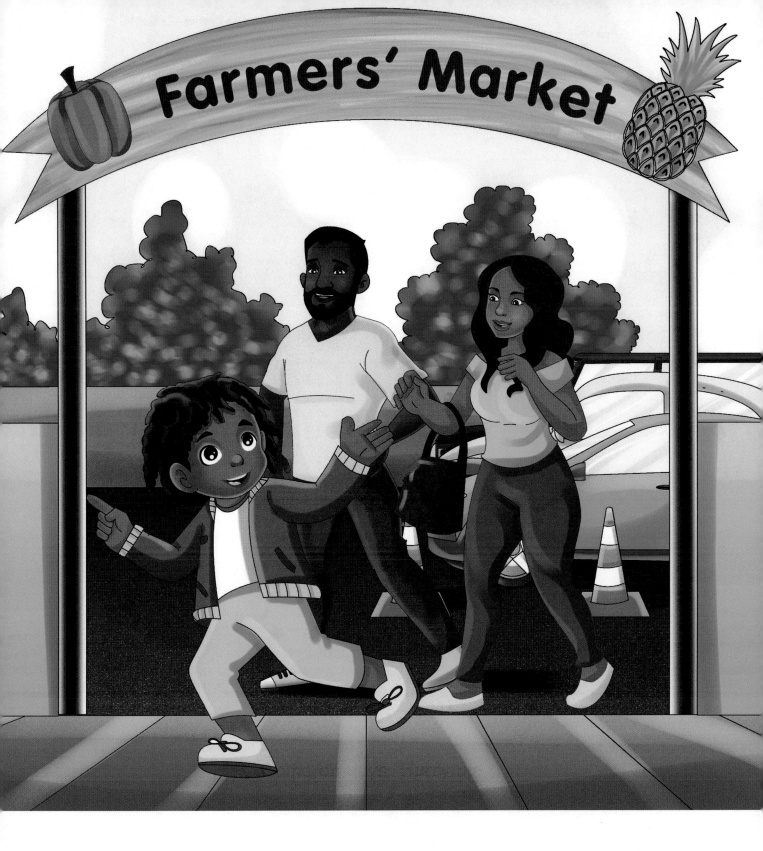

"Come on guys. Hurry up!"

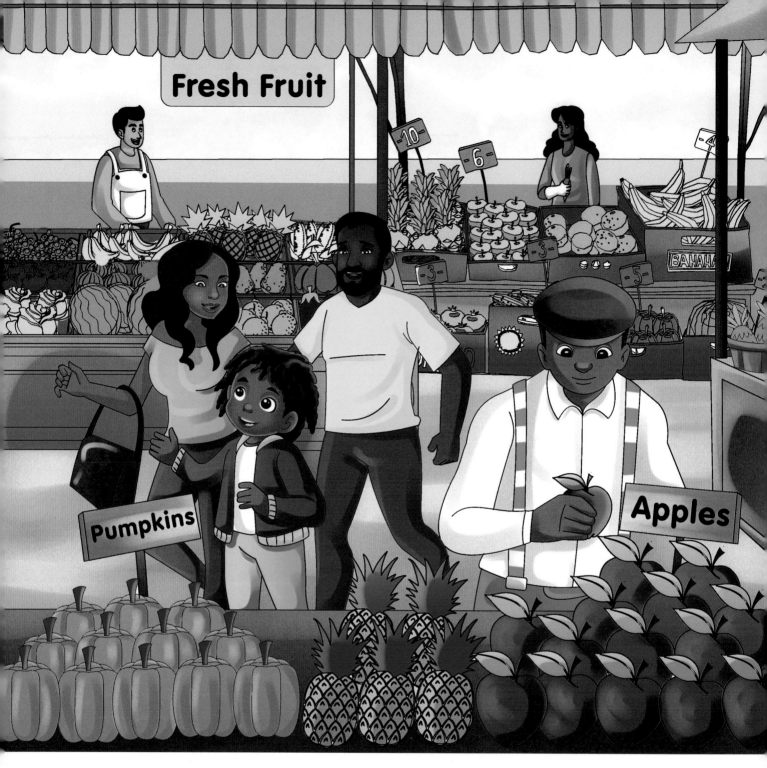

"Every day we should try to eat many different colors of the rainbow," said Rico.

"That's right, Rico. Fruits and vegetables have a lot of nutrients," Mom explained.

"What are nutrients?" Rico asked.

"That's a great question!" Mom declared.

"Nutrients help you to live and grow and be healthy," explained Mom.

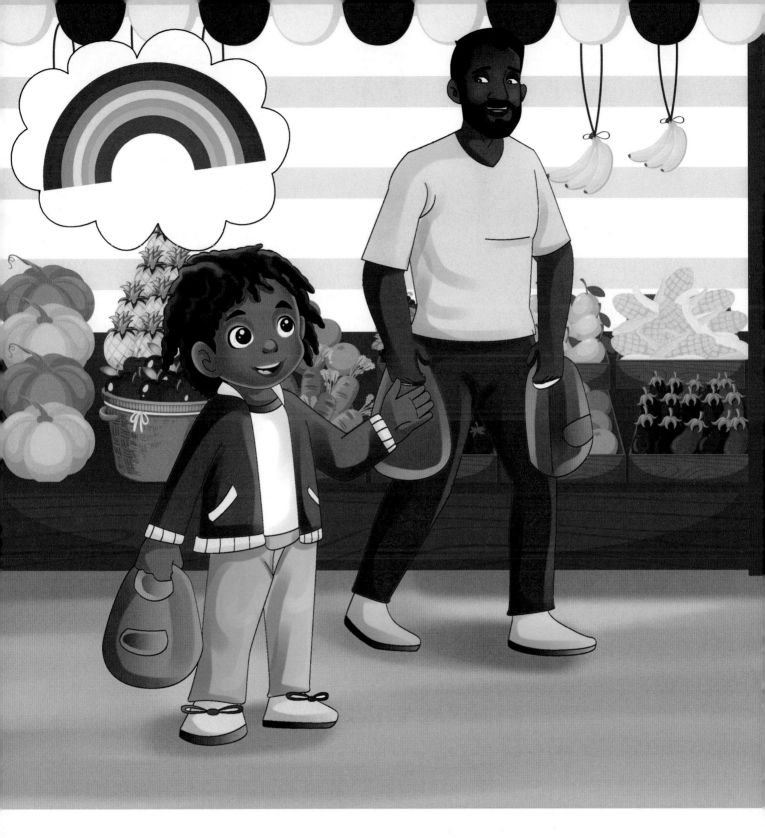

"Do you know the colors of the rainbow, son"?

"Of course, Dad! I learned that when I was little."

"Red is the first color of the rainbow. Let's look for red foods,"
Rico said.

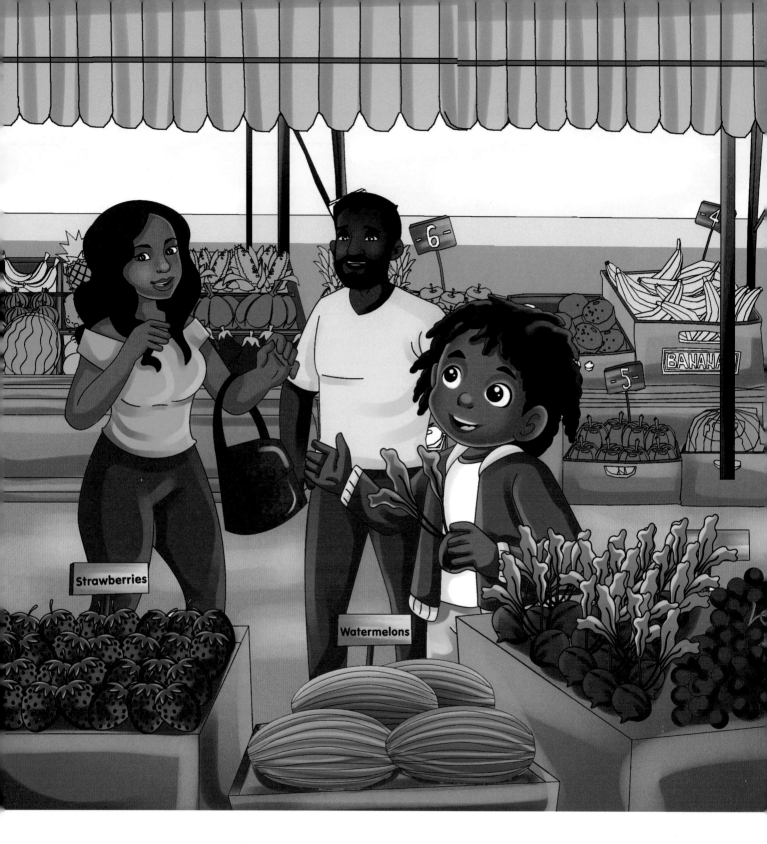

"I like strawberries and watermelon and grapes," said Rico.
"Those three foods are red!"

"Beets are another really healthy red food.
I tried them at Auntie's house and I liked them."

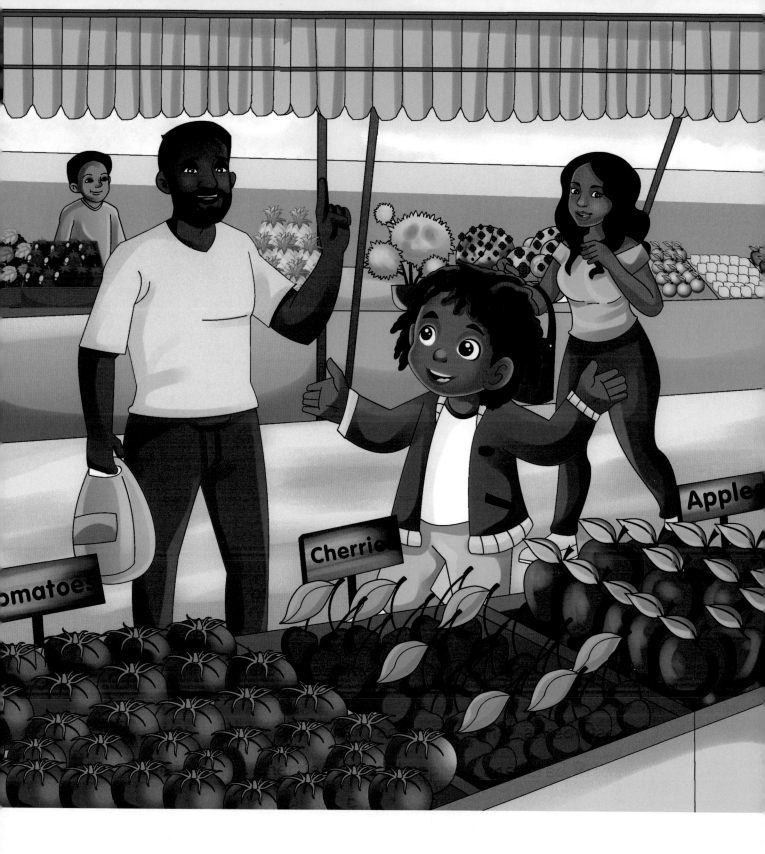

"Can you think of any other red foods, son?" asked Dad.

"Tomatoes . . . cherries . . . red apples," answered Rico.

"Good job, Rico," said Mom.

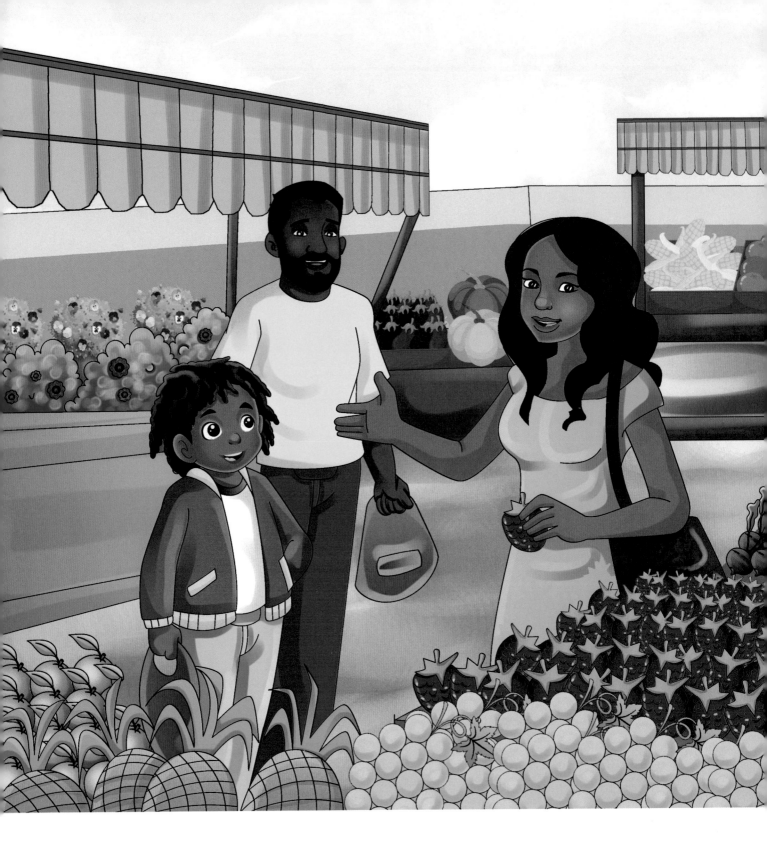

"Don't forget about cranberries and red pears and pomegranates," said Dad.

"And raspberries. Don't forget about the raspberries," said Mom. "Those are my favorites."

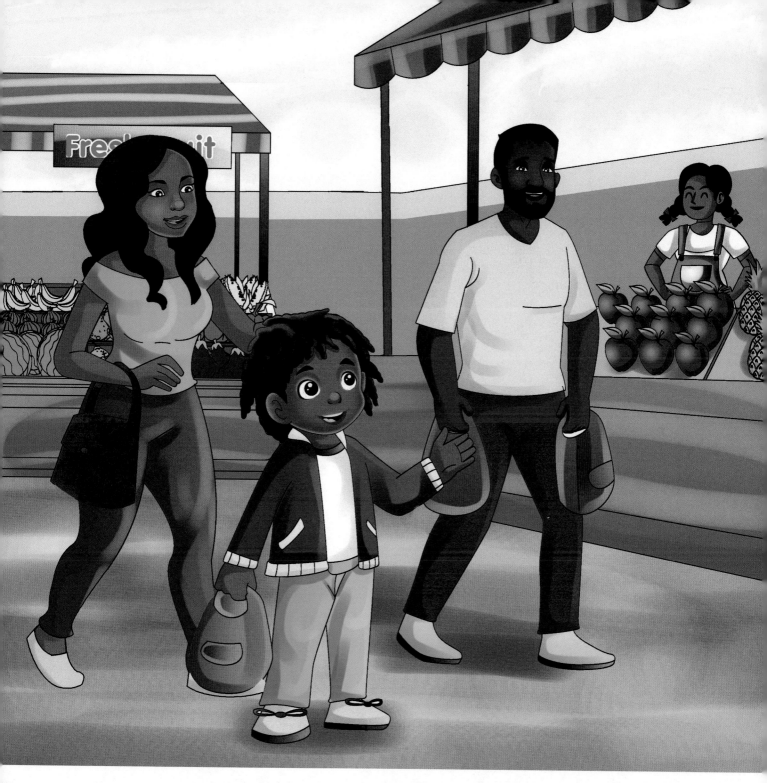

"The next two colors in the rainbow are orange and yellow," said Rico.

"Orange and yellow fruits and vegetables are very healthy," explained Mom.

"Do orange and yellow fruits and vegetables have a lot of nutrients?" Rico asked.

"Yes, they do," Dad answered.

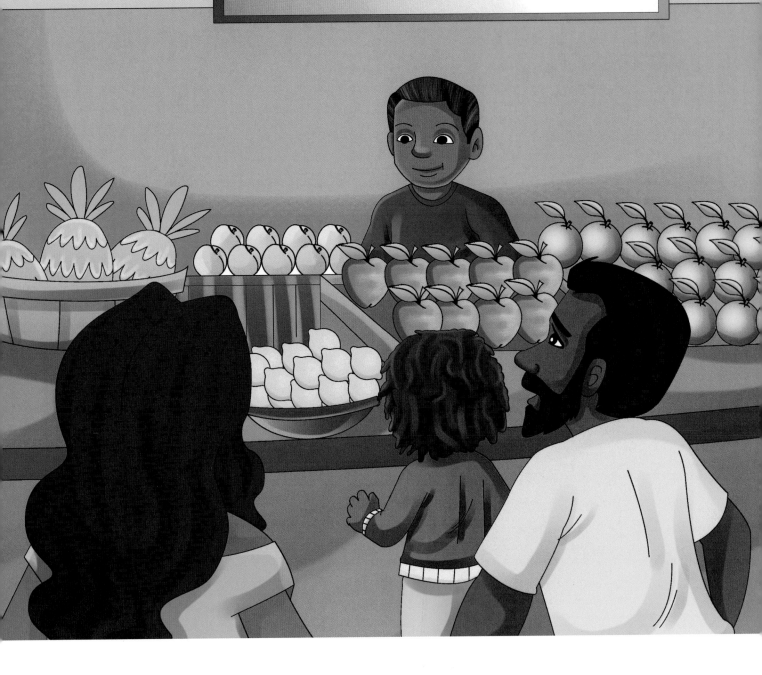

"I see yellow apples and lemons and oranges," said Rico.

"I see nectarines, grapefruit, pineapple, and peaches," said Dad.

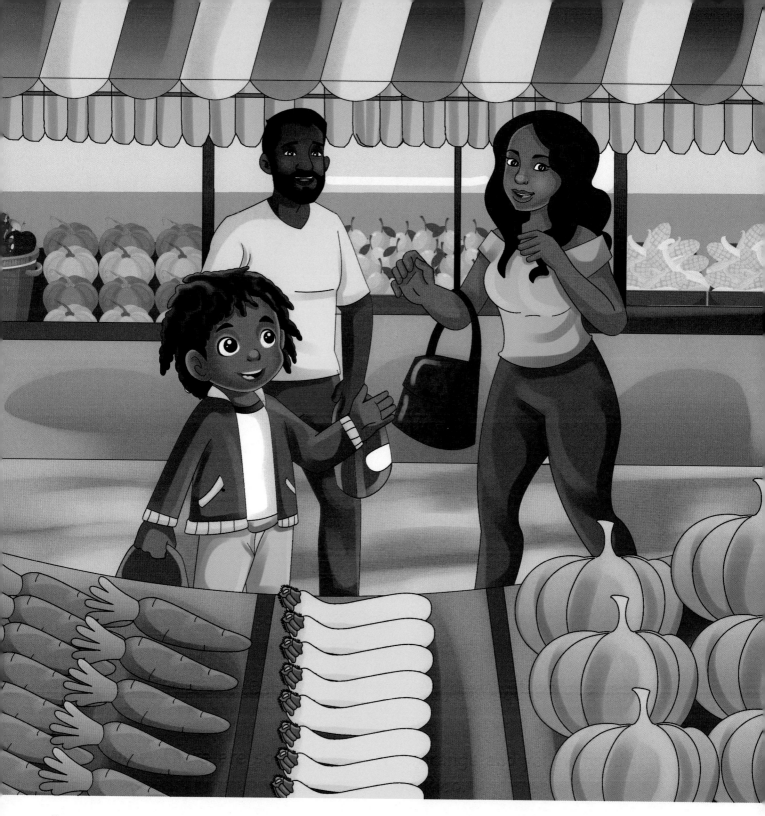

"Look! Over there! I see corn and pumpkins, and squash, and carrots,"
shouted Mom.

"Wow! There are so many different orange and yellow foods
we can eat," said Rico.

These fruits and vegetables are all very healthy food choices,"
said Mom.

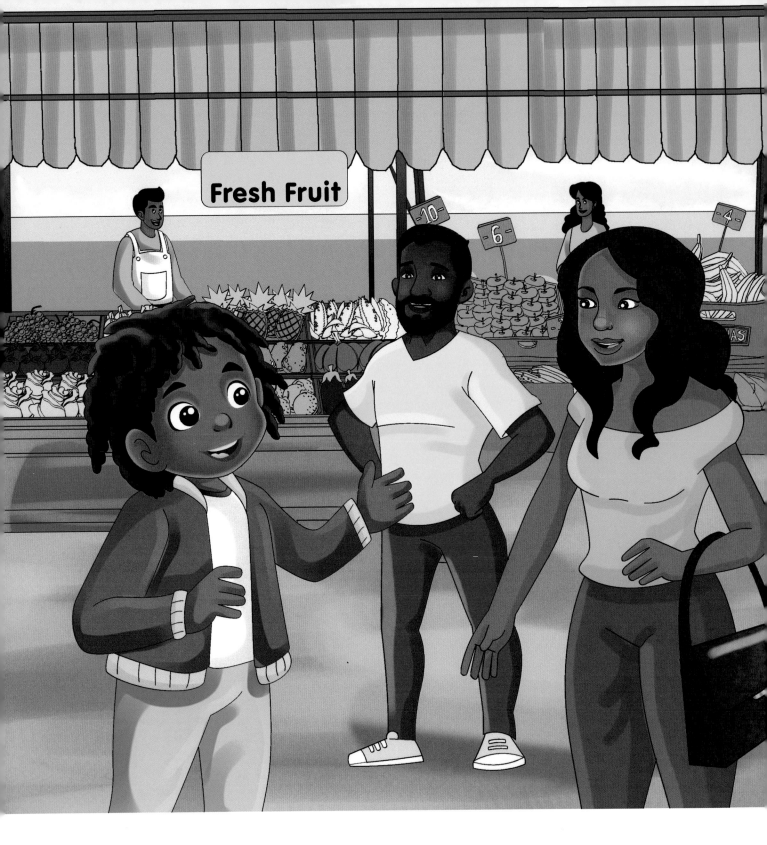

"I know Mom.
It's better to eat fruits and vegetables than to eat foods
that don't have many nutrients," said Rico.

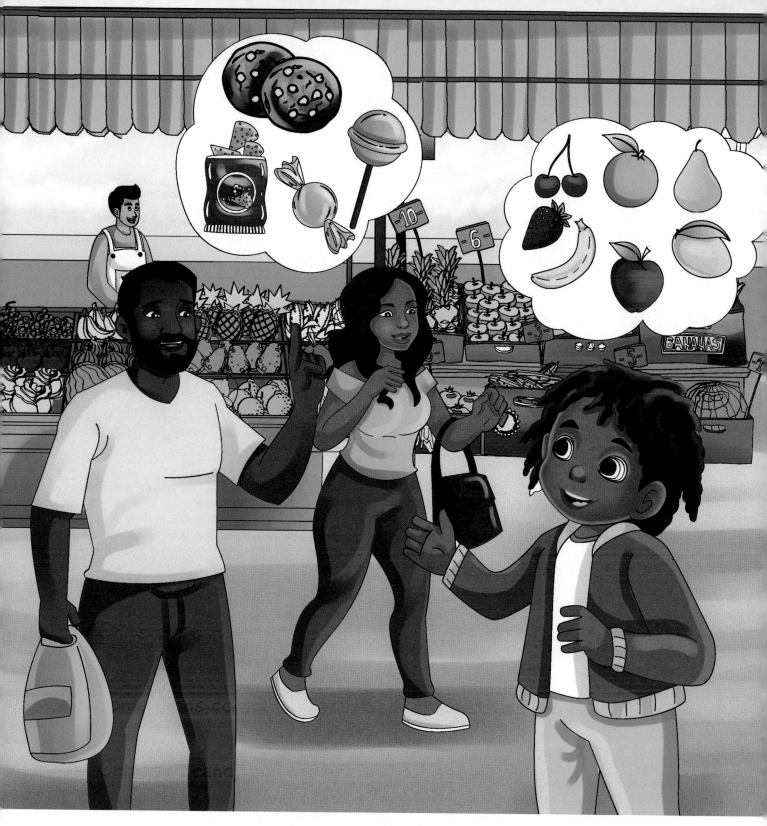

"Some foods do not help your body to be strong and healthy," explained Dad.

"Chips and candy and cookies are not as healthy as fruits and vegetables," said Rico.

"That's right, Rico," Mom agreed.

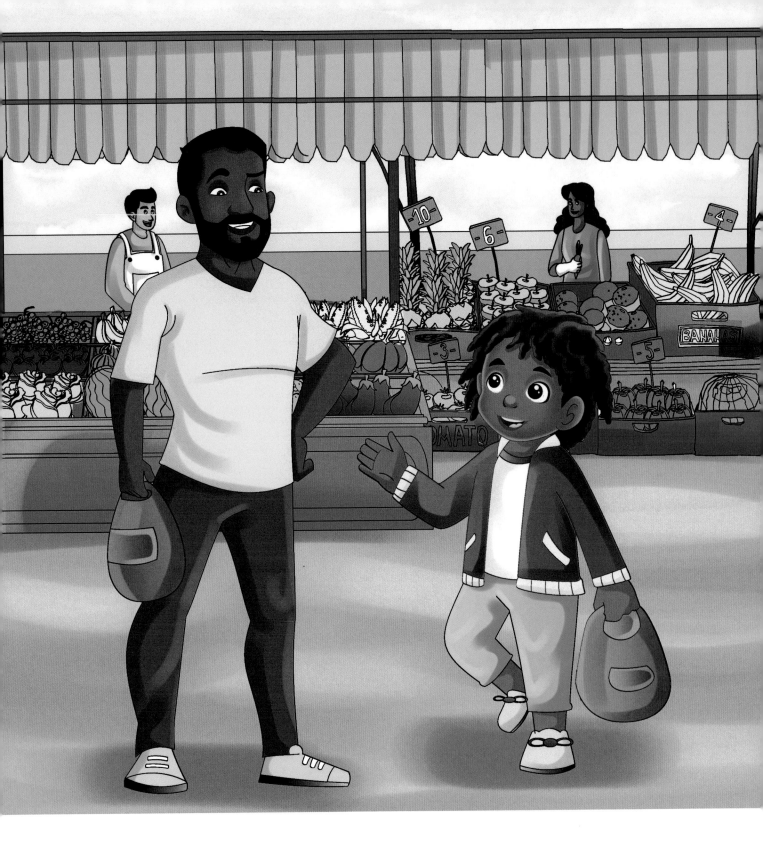

"That's why I always tell you to eat your vegetables," said Dad.

"So I can be healthy!" said Rico.

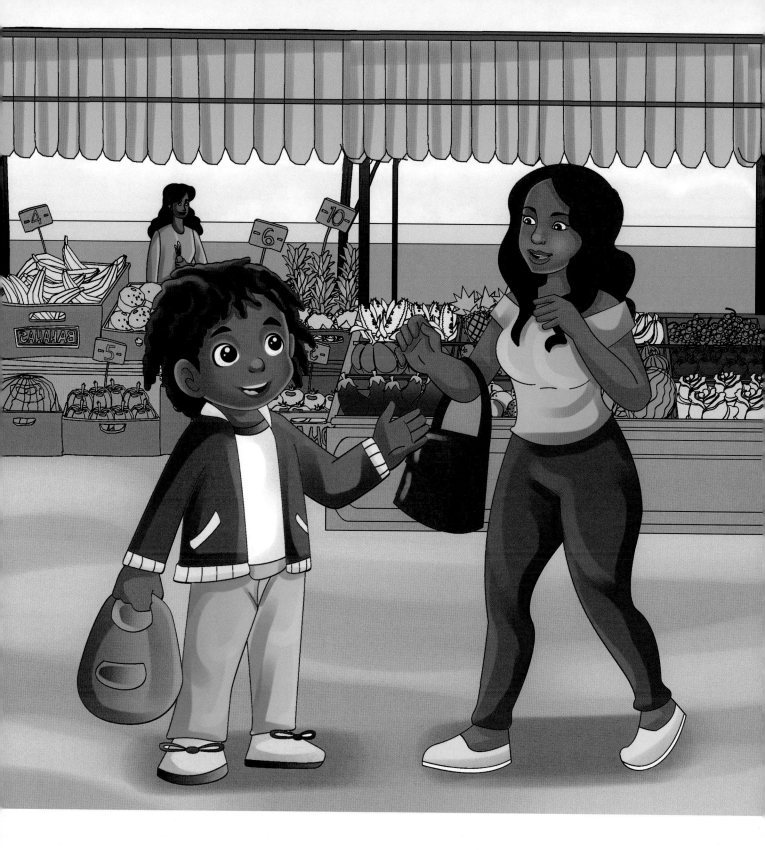

What is the next color in the rainbow?" asked Mom.
"Green!" said Rico.

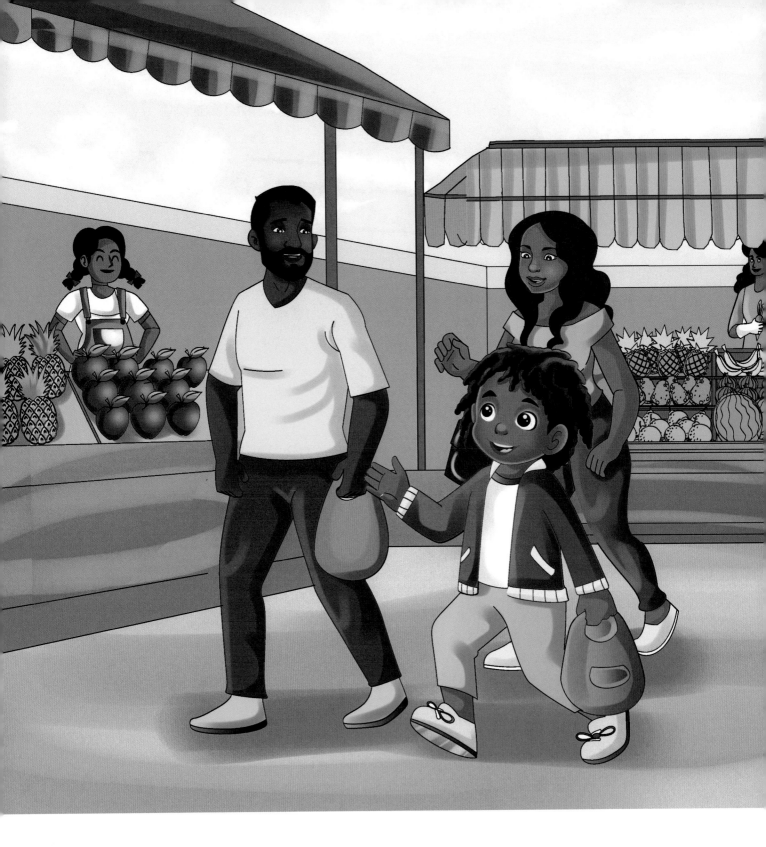

"Well, let's find some green foods. This should be easy,"
said Dad.

"This is really easy. There are so many green vegetables,"
explained Rico.

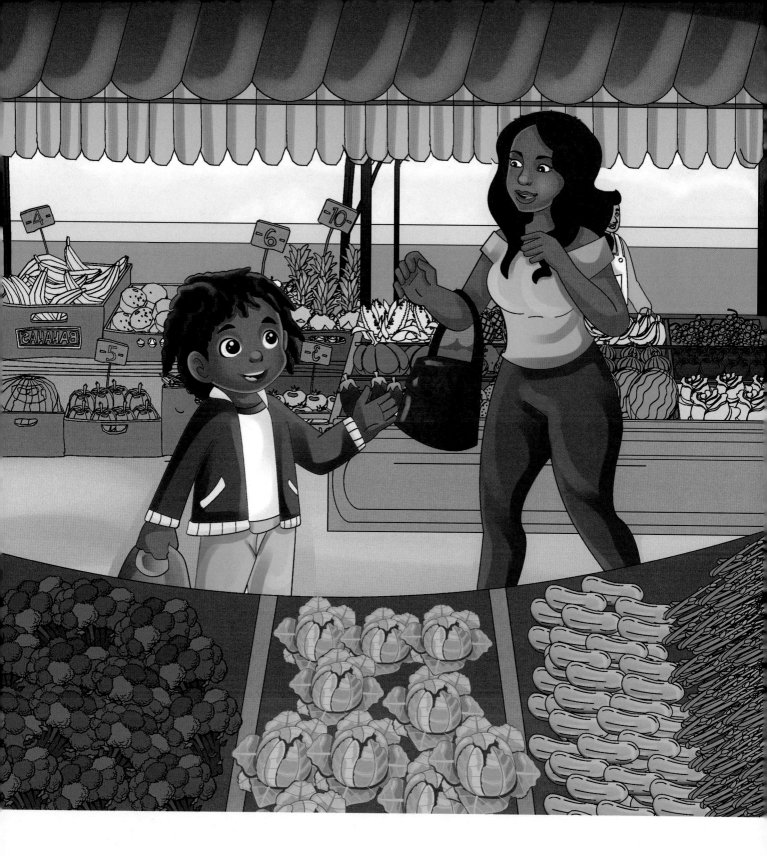

"Broccoli, cabbage, green beans, peas," said Rico.

"Cucumber, celery, and asparagus," said Mom.

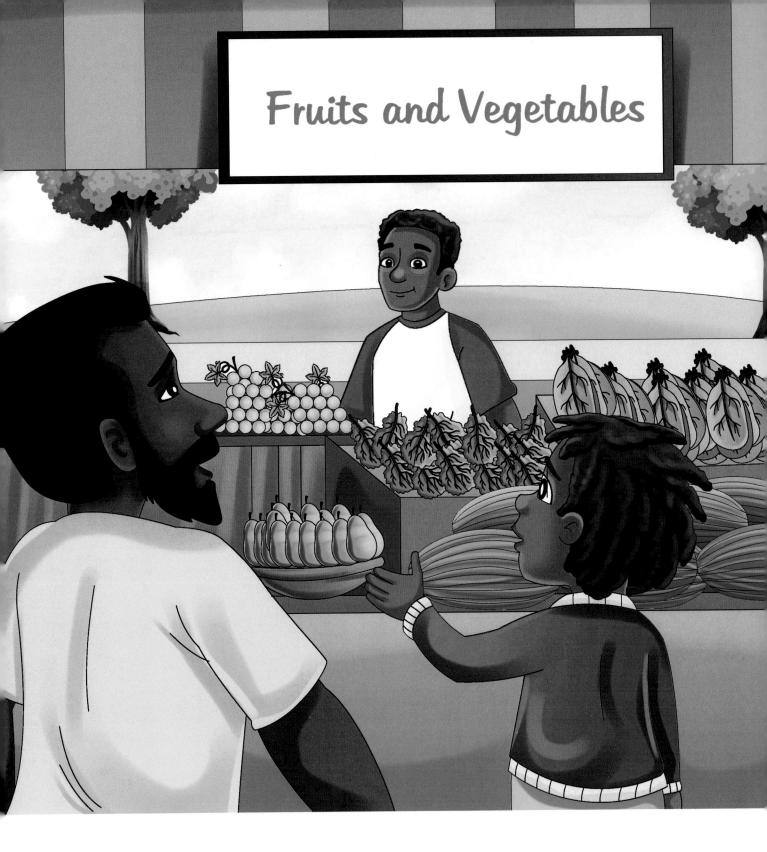

"Avocados, green apples, grapes, and kiwi," said Dad.

"And lettuce and spinach," said Rico.
"I always eat lettuce and spinach when I eat salads."

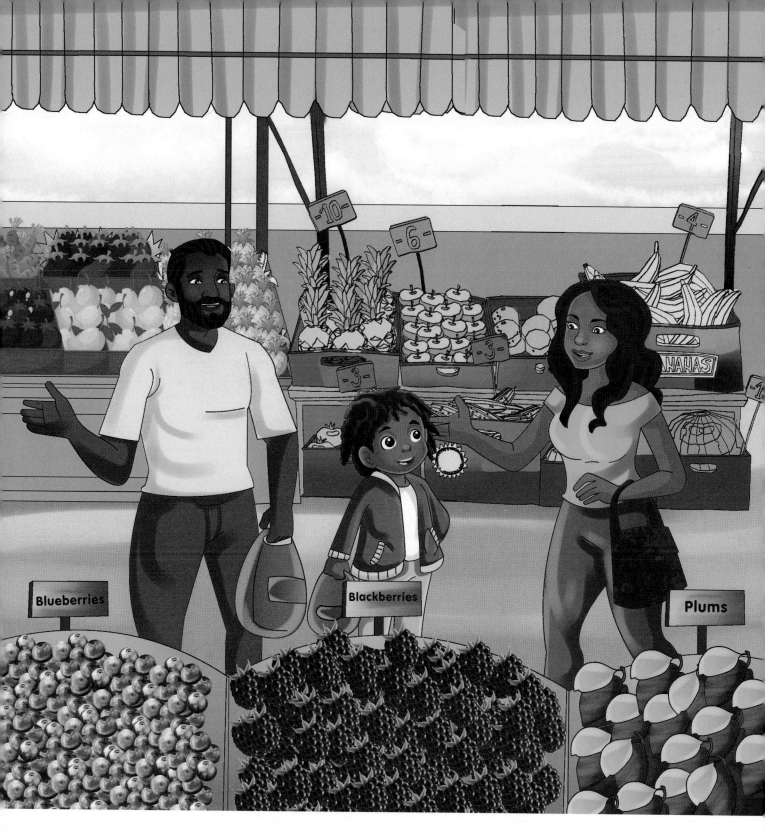

"The rest of the rainbow colors are blue or purple," said Dad.

"I see plums!" said Rico.

"The plums look delicious!" said Mom.

"Blueberries and blackberries are my favorite!" said Dad.

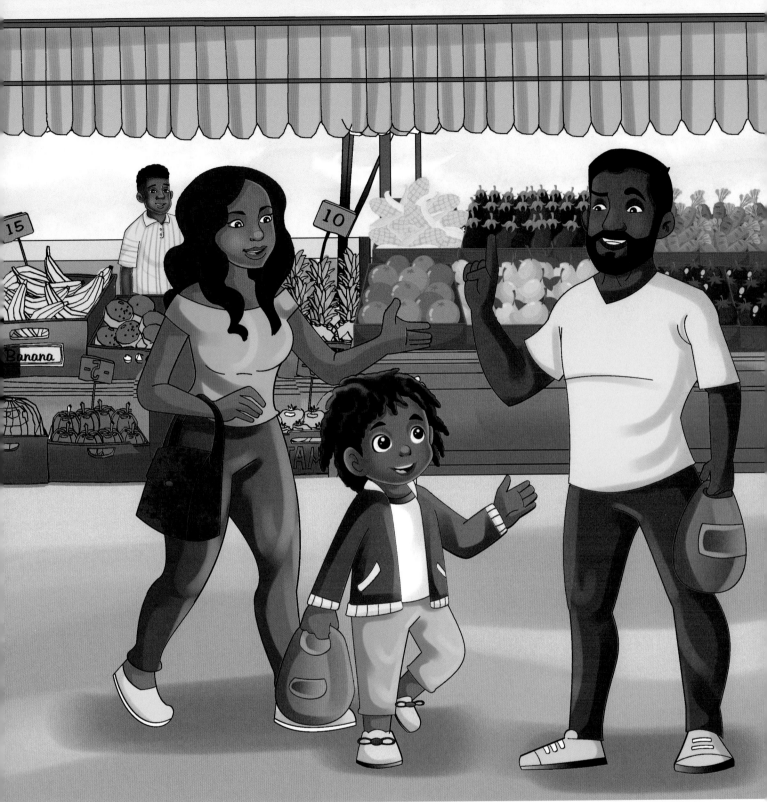

"I ate a lot of different colored foods when I was at Auntie's house. That is why I said 'I "ate a rainbow' " Rico told his parents.

"I see, son," said Dad.

"Eating a rainbow is not actually eating a real rainbow," explained Rico.

"Eating a rainbow is a way of remembering to eat a lot of different color foods so that your body can be strong and healthy," said Mom.

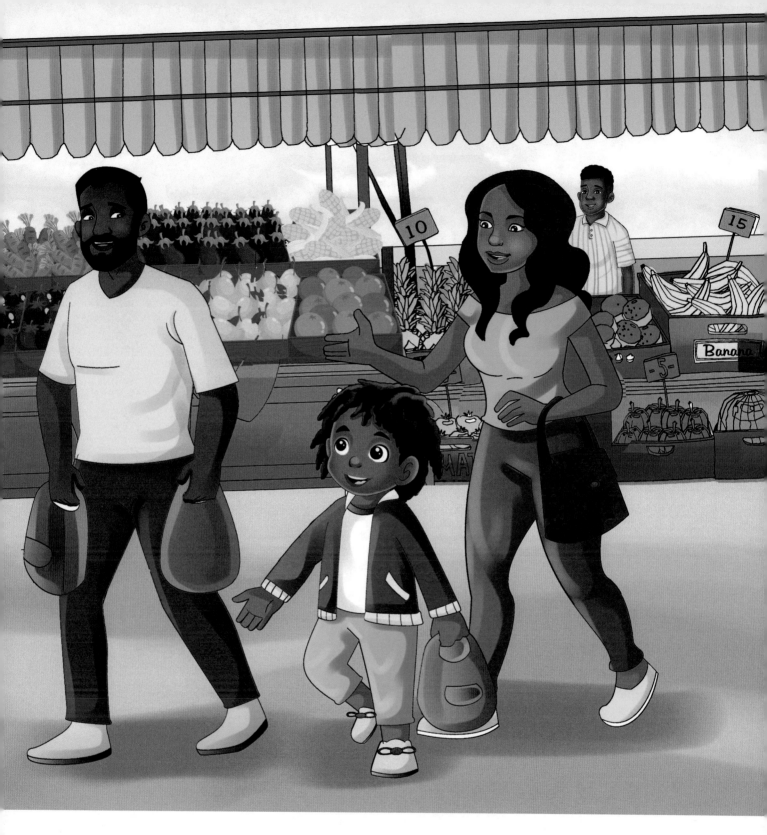

"This was really fun!" said Dad.

"This was a great idea!" said Mom.

Now can we go home and eat our rainbow?" asked Rico.

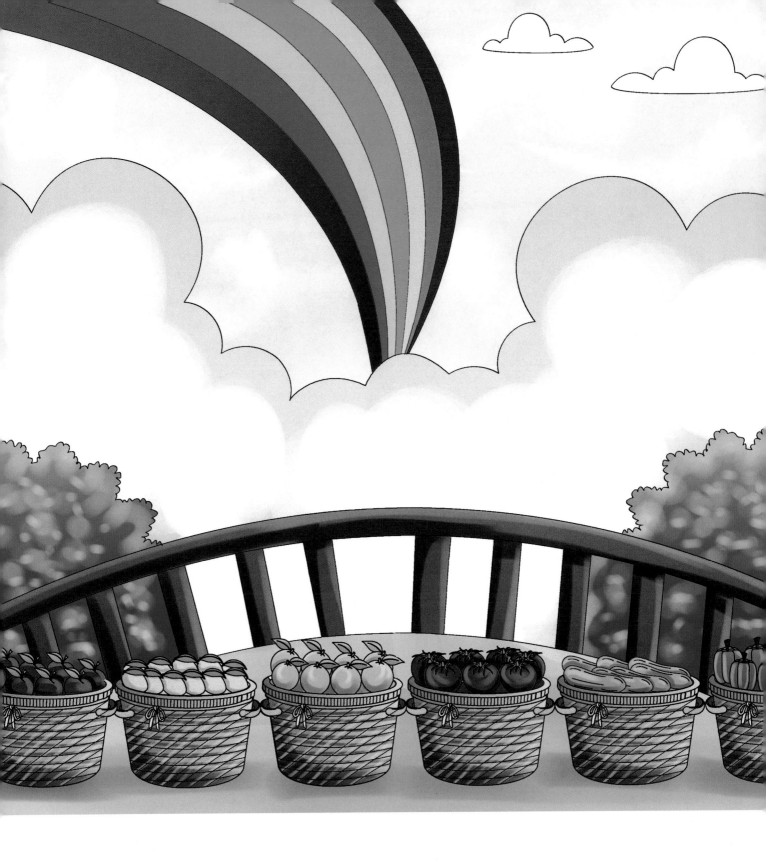

The End

ABOUT THE AUTHOR

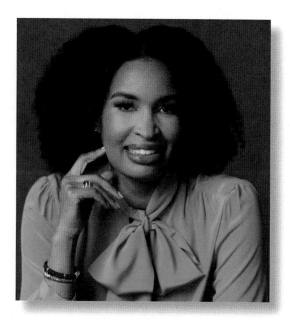

Jessica M. Miller, DrPH believes that introducing children to healthy eating messages at an early age is one of the most important ways to build a bright future for a child. She developed her interest in health and wellness campaigns as a junior high school assistant principal, where the food choices of teens and pre-teens fueled a sincere passion for spreading knowledge and shaping positive change.

As a curious child growing up in Detroit, Michigan, Jessica fell in love with reading as a way to imagine new places and see the world differently. The Sweet Pickles children's book series was her first book subscription, which stimulated an early habit of reading. She hopes her book will help children find their own joy in reading and inspire a lifetime of healthy habits.

Jessica obtained her Doctor of Public Health degree in health education from Loma Linda University. She works as a public health specialist, conducting research and evaluation of health services and community programs and as an adjunct professor of public health sciences.

With more than 20 years of education experience and a love for children, Jessica has a Master of Arts degree in education and is credentialed through the State of California as a teacher and administrator.

Jessica lives in Southern California and enjoys traveling, reading, and a variety of outdoor leisure activities.

Join Jessica at RicoEatsARainbow on Facebook and Instagram.

Email: RicoEatsARainbow@gmail.com

AFTERWORD

You've just finished a glorious trip into Rico's rainbow of fruits and vegetables so juicy and alive. You wish they could jump off the page into your mouth!

Even vegetable haters find it hard to resist the vibrantly colored illustrations, which makes Rico's journey fascinating and appealing.

Between the pages of *Rico Eats a Rainbow* is an urgent call for parents, by their words and examples, to tackle the biggest health challenge facing our children today - childhood obesity. In the United States, approximately 17% of children aged 2 – 19 years are obese. An additional 15% are overweight.

Childhood obesity can propel children down a path of health problems that were once considered adult health problems: Type 2 diabetes, high blood pressure, and high cholesterol. Likewise, obesity can affect all aspects of children, including leading to poor self-esteem and depression.

Through the lens of her nephew Rico, author Jessica Miller, DrPH pens a wonderful story to help parents and educators talk with children about adopting healthy eating habits.

Dr. Miller, a public health professional, health education advocate, and former school principal, recalls school cafeteria scenes of children guzzling sugary drinks and lunchboxes stuffed with salty snacks and other nutrient lacking foods that put children on a dangerous path to childhood and adult obesity.

This book is great on so many levels as it lays the foundation for our children to develop a healthy lifestyle by healthy eating; it does so in a way that children understand. When coupled with regular exercise, this message will help children to be on the path to good health.

Food and culture are interwoven. *Rico Eats a Rainbow* serves up an inspiring message: Food is meant to be explored. It's the ingredient that brings us together. Pull up a chair; take a taste.

Ernest Levister, Jr. M.D. F.A.C.P., F.A.C.P.M
Former Clinical Professor of Internal & Occupational Medicine
University of California Irvine